D1564503

Viagra

The Ultimate Guide to Use Viagra Pills to Cure Erectile Dysfunction, Premature Ejaculation, Increase Libido, Last Longer and Enjoy an Endless Sexual Experience

Dr. John Smith

PUBLISHED BY:
Green Book Publishing LTD

24 Tax Suite 137 B Westlink House 981 Great West Road
Brentford, United Kingdom, TW8 9DN

First Print 2022

Green Book Publishing ®

1. Everything about Viagra

Pfizer, Inc., a pharmaceutical corporation, launched Viagra, the first oral therapeutic treatment for male impotence, in the year 1998. Viagra is the registered name of the drug. It a drug that fits into the category of phosphodiesterase-5 inhibitors. This medication is also known by its chemical name, which is sildenafil citrate.

Where can Viagra be Purchased?

Erectile dysfunction (ED) can be treated with prescription medications like Viagra, which is a brand name for the drug. If you have ED, you won't be capable to get or sustain an erection. Viagra is authorized for use in this manner in guys who are at least 18 years old.

Sildenafil citrate is the principal constituent in this drug. PDE5i are the category of drugs that this one is classified under. Sildenafil achieves its effects by enhancing blood-stream to the penis, which makes it much simpler to have and keep an erection. Nonetheless, in order for this medicine to operate, the consumer should be first sexually excited.

Sildenafil is accessible in tablets to be gulped. It is recommended to take it around one hour before engaging in sexual activity; nevertheless, it may be assumed from 30 minutes to 4 hours ahead. 3 different dosage levels are available for Sildenafil: 25mg, 50mg, and 100mg.

Where did the concept for its creation come from?

The strong love pill was first created to soothe the symptoms of a different kind of physical discomfort; it was not intended to do the passionate job it does now, which is to give millions of men a lift.

In 1985, chemists laboring for Pfizer named Albert Wood and Peter Dunn came up with the idea for a medication that would later be known as sildenafil citrate. They believed that it might be useful in bringing down excessive blood pressure as well as treating angina. Pfizer's small blue thrill pill was just the beginning of what would ultimately become the world's first consumable elixir for erectile dysfunction. Unbeknownst to them, they were sitting on the heart of what would be transformed into the most famous oral elixir.

Pfizer initiated clinical tests of the medication, which by that time had been given the trade name Viagra, in the early 1990s in the country of Britain. Apparently, it appeared like anything amazing would happen during the testing. After that, an odd and unanticipated turn of events began to take place. The participants in the study started reporting some pretty unusual adverse effects, some of which were quite intriguing.

Viagra wasn't as fruitful as scientists had aspired it would be in dealing with cardiovascular illnesses, but it was incredibly effective at something else as well. It was opening up the capillaries and arteries in the penis and filling penile tissue with blood.

In other words, it caused males to work extremely hard (in other places besides the fields), often for up to four hours in a row. People didn't want to return the prescription because one of its negative effects was experiencing erections that were stronger, more stable, and lasted longer than usual.

The researchers were aware that they were sitting on a potentially game-changing discovery. They had produced some very potent substance, powerful enough to restore youth and vitality to middle-aged men in as little as thirty to sixty minutes after swallowing the pill (on average). Pfizer promptly abandoned their plans to test Viagra as a heart medication and shifted their focus to developing the drug as a treatment for erectile dysfunction after they realized they were on to something groundbreaking.

In 1993, research began to investigate whether or not Viagra could be used as a treatment for erectile dysfunction. They consisted of around 3,000 patients going from 20 to 85. It was demonstrated to be effective in 21 separate trials, each of which was conducted independently.

A significant patent for the game-changing medication was finally awarded to the multinational pharmaceutical company headquartered in New York City in 1996. The FDA gave the consent to the drug to be utilized as a therapy for impotence on March 27, 1998. This was the company's next significant victory on its path to bringing the product to market.

It was from that location when the dams broke open. The novel diamond-shaped doozie was in high demand across the United States, and pharmacists had a hard time keeping up with public demand for it. According to the Los Angeles Times, the new medication set a record during its first week on the market for the number of prescriptions that were written for it. It is estimated that 40,000 prescriptions for Viagra were filled in just the first few weeks when the drug was available to the public.

When everything was said and done, this was the largest launch of a medicine in the history of the world.

The enthusiasm that was produced by the revolutionary virility enhancer has soon reached a boiling point. Even in places where Viagra is not yet available, Newsweek described it as the "hottest new medicine in history" in an article entitled "The Globe is Crazy for Viagra".

The publisher of Penthouse welcomed it as a manly wonder drug that would "release the American male libido" from the clutches of feminists who tried to "emasculate" them. A senior columnist for Playboy predicted that the contentious prescription would be "as important as the birth-control pill."

By the year 2001, Viagra had become a truly ubiquitous phenomenon all over the world. The drug's annual sales soared above the $1 billion mark, making it one of the biggest lucrative prescription drugs that Pfizer has ever developed.

Some people believe the word Viagra was chosen because it alludes to a man's virility and vitality. Others contend that the fact that it rhymes with the powerful waterfalls of Niagara is not a coincidence and that it was deliberate. Pfizer isn't revealing it. Even with insurance coverage, the cost of one pill can range anywhere from $34 to $40, making it far from an affordable form of entertainment.

Not bad for a little medication that was once developed to alleviate chest discomfort.

Mechanism of Action of Viagra

When you become aroused, your body secretes nitric oxide down below. Nitric oxide is a chemical that sets off the chain of events that is critical for an erection. However, an enzyme (protein) known as Phosphodiesterase type 5 (PDE5) degrades specific messengers that are involved in this process, so blocking the effect that is wanted to occur.

PDE5 inhibitors, such as Viagra, are frequently employed as a treatment option for erectile dysfunction (ED), which refers to the inability of a man to achieve or keep an erection. Impotence can arise from many different elements.

Viagra for men and other medications for erectile dysfunction (ED) like Cialis (tadalafil) and Levitra (vardenafil) operate by assisting in the relaxation of muscles and arteries located within the penis. This enables a raise in the quantity of sap that is capable to arrive at the penis. Only when aroused does the mix of relaxation and increased blood flow assist swell the penis. You are capable to have and sustain an erection in this manner.

How quickly do you feel the effects?

You can take Viagra anywhere from thirty minutes to four hours before you want to engage in sexual activity, as the medication swiftly enters your system after you take it and begins to work after about an hour, but the optimal timing is thirty minutes.

Because of this, you should take it approximately one hour before engaging in sexual activity; nevertheless, there is a larger window of time during which you can still obtain the benefits of the medication. However, you need to be aroused in order for it to operate, as was said earlier.

You could be wondering if there are any methods that can assist the prescription work even faster, such as chewing the tablet, smashing it, or dissolving it under your tongue. On the other hand, this isn't how it's supposed to operate, so you have to take it all at once.

Viagra action time

The effects of Viagra can last from 3 to 7 hours, and it can vary from the individual who takes it and the amount they use. Actually, there is a chance that some people will experience many erections during this time frame. In contrast, the event that the drug can persist in your organism for up to 6 hours does not necessarily assure that your erection will continue for that period of time.

In fact, you should seek immediate medical attention if your erection continues for more than three hours, regardless of whether or not it is uncomfortable. A disorder known as priapism is diagnosed when an erection continues for at least three hours straight. This condition has the potential to cause irreversible harm to the tissue that helps you get an erection.

It is more likely that you will have a prolonged erection if you have sickle cell anemia, multiple myeloma, leukemia or certain penile abnormalities (such Peyronie's disease).

How should I assume it for maximum benefits?

Here are a few pointers for using Viagra in a way that is both safe and effective:

Always adhere to the approved and safe dosages

When treating erectile dysfunction (ED), the typical suggested dose of Viagra is 50 milligrams (mg), although your doctor may prescribe anything from 25 mg to 100 mg instead.

It is suggested to use the medication no more than one time per day. This indicates that you shouldn't take a pill each time you engage in sexual activity during the course of the day if you plan on engaging in sexual activity more than once. Also, if you take a pill and it doesn't work for you, you shouldn't try to make it work twice as hard by taking another tablet. If you take more Viagra than the doctor prescribed, you could put yourself at risk for significant side effects.

Because Viagra might have side effects on other regions of the body, such as the heart and lungs, it is essential to take the medication exactly how your doctor prescribes and follow all of their recommendations. In addition, if the dosage that was recommended to you isn't effective, they may make some changes in order to discover one that is.

Take it with no food in your stomach

Viagra can be taken with or without food, although studies have shown that it works significantly better when taken on an empty stomach. Therefore, in order to get the most out of it, you should try to take it on an empty stomach.

If you do find yourself eating before you take the medication, however, you should try to avoid taking it with a meal that is high in fat because this can slow down the rate at which the medication is absorbed and the speed with which it begins to work.

Some Important Information to Remember Before Taking Viagra

Viagra is not for every man, nor should it be taken by every man

Before beginning this medication, you should consult your physician if you are currently using nitrates, if you suffer from chest pain or low blood pressure, if you have recently suffered a heart attack, heart failure, or stroke, or if you had of any of these problems in the past. Viagra can cause adverse reactions in patients who take certain medications or who have certain health conditions; therefore, it is imperative that you inform your physician of all the medications that you currently use in addition to informing them of any allergies you may have.

Timing issues

It is important to wait at least two hours after your previous meal before taking the tablet, so make sure to schedule enough time in advance. The recommended time to have the dose is 1 hour earlier than an intercourse. You have ONLY to assume the dose ONCE per day.

Viagra efficacy can be reduced depending on the foods you eat and the times you eat them

On days that you intend to take Viagra, try to stay away from foods that are high in fat. Because of this, the effects of Viagra may take longer to manifest. Before you take Viagra, you should try to spread out your heavier meals throughout the day and not have heavy meals that contain high-fat foods like flesh, oily aliments, and other high-fat ingredients.

Viagra comes in different doses

Although Viagra is available in pills of 25, 50, and 100 milligrams, the recommended starting dose you should take is 50 milligrams. It will depend on your condition whether or not your physician will suggest that you assume a higher or lower dosage of the medication. The highest dose that is recommended is 100 milligrams (mg).

There is no guarantee that the first dose of Viagra will be effective

Viagra is not a magic pill; in order to achieve an erection, it must be combined with sexual activation, and using it for the first time may not be successful. It is recommended that you give it at least two to three tries before deciding whether or not it is working for you. If you are concerned that it is not going to work while you are with your partner, you should first attempt to take it on your own and stimulate yourself. It may also be beneficial to stimulate the penis directly after taking the tablet in order to achieve the desired results.

2. Functioning of the Penile Erection

P enis blood vessels relax and dilate to allow blood to fill them when a man is sexually excited. An erection is the result of blood becoming entrapped in a small space at a high pressure. The central nervous system is liable for the reflex action of ejaculation.

Anatomy

It is composed of:

Organs that have two chambers termed the corpora cavernosa that run the length of the organ and are filled with cavernous blood vessels (like a sponge).

Underside of the corpora cavernosa, where the urethra or tube for urine and sperm runs.

There are two major arteries and various veins and nerves around the urethra.

The rod of the penis that is the longest section of it.
At the end of the shaft, there we find the glans.

How does a man get an erection?

A rush of blood rushes through the cavernous arteries when the corpora cavernosa relax and dilate. An erection is formed as a result of the blood being trapped under high pressure.

Sensory and cerebral stimulation is necessary before an erection can occur. Nerve signals stimulate the penis during sexual desire. The corpora cavernosa relaxes as a result of stimuli from the central nervous system and regional veins, permitting the blood to enter and replenish the open areas. Pressure in the corpora cavernosa results in an erection due to the expansion of the penis.

Keeping the erection strong requires blood to be trapped within the corpora cavernosa, which the tunica albuginea does. As the muscles of the penis stiffen, bloodstream to the penis is halted and outflow channels are unclosed, reversing erectile dysfunction.

What is the cause of this?

The most common cause is sexual arousal, which can be triggered by something you see, feel, or simply think about. It is also probable for erections to happen randomly. "Spontaneous Erects" is the term for these sporadic erections. Slug documentaries aren't exactly known for their sexual content, so don't be alarmed when you find yourself experiencing a stiffy while viewing one. Even if you didn't have a sex dream, it's typical to wake up with the morning wood.

Erectile Dysfunction: The Science Behind the Myth

A condition known as impotence (or erectile dysfunction) is the incapacity to obtain and maintain an erection strong enough for sexual activity.

It's not usually a reason for alarm if you occasionally have erection problems. It can bring to stressful thoughts and impact your self-esteem, and even lead to relationship issues. The chance of heart problems in men increases when they have difficulty strengthening or maintaining an erection.

What induce an erection?

Problems with erection might lead to ED at any point in life. Enhanced blood flow to the penis is the cause of the erection. Thoughts of sexual activity or making physical contact with one's penis are typically more effective at increasing the bloodstream.

Whenever a man experiences sexual arousal, one of the muscles that is located within the arteries in the penis softens. As a result, the penile arteries and the two chambers within the penis can receive more blood. The penis stiffens when blood fills the chambers.

Is ED a common problem?

A study by medical researchers estimates that 28 million Americans have trouble with ED. ED is more frequent with advancing age. Mild to severe erectile dysfunction affects 10 percent more males each decade of life, according to research from the University of Pennsylvania. To cite an instance, more than 50% of men in their 50s may be affected by ED at some point in their lives.

ED, on the other hand, can strike people as young as twenty-five. As stated by a study conducted in 2012, ¼ of males searching for treatment for erectile dysfunction is under 38. When compared to older men, these individuals had a higher rate of ED and higher rates of smoking and drug use. Young men's lifestyle choices may play a role in their risk of developing ED.

Age-related erectile dysfunction is more common, however it is not unavoidable. Overall, a healthy lifestyle improves your sexual performance.

If you have diabetes, working with your doctor to keep your blood sugar levels in check is essential. Preventing ED can be done by limiting the damage that can be done. Investigate the link between erectile dysfunction and type 2 diabetes.

"Peyronie's" Disease Penile Erection

What is the Peyronie's disease?

Cicatrix tissue in the penis can lead it to fold, incline, or shrink as a result of Peyronie's disease. When the cicatrix tissue (plaque) is forming, you may experience pain in a specific area of your penis. This pain is caused by the cicatrix tissue. You can fold your penis up, down, or to the side when erect depending on the placement of the cicatrix. A recessed or "hourglass" shape is more common in men with this issue than a visible curvature.

Men's erections are rarely precisely straight. Peyronie's disease is not necessarily indicated by a slight curvature of the penis. The condition known as Peyronie's disease does not affect men who have always had a bend in their penises.

When the penis becomes erect, is it common for the cicatrix to form uppermost, forcing it to curve upright. If the cicatrix is on the downside, your penis will curve earthward; if the cicatrix is on the lateral part of the penis, it will curve laterally. This might cause the penis to become "smaller" if the cicatrix expands above or below the shaft simultaneously. Occasionally, the scar will go around the penis completely, narrowing it down to the size of an hourglass in the middle. Some men with this illness may develop scar tissue that feels like bone because of the calcium in it.

What exactly is the function of the penis?

Urine and sperm are both carried by your penis. The urethral canal that takes urine from the blister to the penis, and the two ducts known as the corpora cavernosa, which replenish with blood in order to have an erection, are all located inside the penis. The tunica albuginea, a strong fibrous sheath, connects all three. It is possible to penetrate your penis when you are having intercourse because of the blood flow to your penis. After orgasm, semen is expelled from the urethra. Ejaculation is the name given to this procedure.

However, urination and ejaculation are unaffected by Peyronie's disease, which affects only the penis.

Peyronie's illness progresses in stages. What are they?

Acute and chronic Peyronie's disease are both forms of the disease.

Between five and fourteen months, this is the acute period. It's during this time that you'll notice a curvature or other change to the contour of your penis. In some cases, your penis may hurt when it's erect or soft.

The curvature in the penis does not worsen in this period since the scar has ceased to grow. When talking about erections, the pain is usually gone by this point, although there are some exceptions. In addition, erectile dysfunction (ED) or difficulties in obtaining or maintaining a hardened penis may arise.

Why are Peyronie disease and penile curvature different?

Peyronie's disease, a type of penile curvature that affects adults, is one of the most common forms of this condition. Congenital penile curvature, also known as chordee, occurs in some males at birth. Mainly, it is not originated by scar tissue and does not get better with time. When a man begins to have more regular erections after puberty, it may not be immediately apparent.

In this disease, erectile function is impaired

When the penis is erect in Peyronie's disease, the scar tissue does not extend, causing the penis to bend or become deformed and possibly painful.

There are some guys who develop Peyronie's disease without any apparent harm. Peyronie's disease can be linked to a genetic trait or other conditions, according to researchers.

Erectile Dysfunction and Benign Prostatic Hyperplasia Treatment with Viagra: How to Use It

The aging process affects every component of the human body. As time passes, many men have both lower erections and enlarged prostates. Male infertility (male erectile dysfunction) and benign prostatic hyperplasia (BPH) are two distinct conditions that grow increasingly prevalent as men age. BPH and ED have traditionally had different approaches to therapy, even though medicinal and surgical approaches to BPH can sometimes result in ED. However, studies have shown that the most popular and effective ED medications can significantly lessen the symptoms of BPH.

A gain of six times in the bloodstream of the penis is required for an erection to occur. Erections are made possible by nitric oxide, a molecule that opens up the arteries of the penis, allowing more blood to flow through and increasing excitement.

A proper erection necessitates the presence of nitric oxide; however, it is not the sole cause of this. cGMP, which enhances the bloodstream to your penis, is produced as a result of this signaling to your artery cells. When talking about PDE-5, the penis produces an organic substance that discomposes cGMP.

A hard erection and an end to the erection are the result of the penis' ability to create cGMP and PDE-5, respectively, during proper ejaculation. A malfunctioning of this complex mechanism occurs in a lot of men suffering from erectile dysfunction, and the use of sildenafil (through Viagra, Levitra, or Cialis) can correct this. PDE-5 is inhibited by all ED medications, allowing more cGMP to enter the bloodstream, resulting in stronger, longer-lasting erections in around 75% of men with ED.

Tablets are generally secure and accepted in the treatment of erectile dysfunction. Painful and long-lasting erections can occur in a small number of cases (priapism). They can also reduce blood pressure because of the dilating action of other arteries in your body. As a result, men who are on an anti-nitrate medicine should avoid using erectile dysfunction pills, and those suffering from ED who are taking alpha blockers for benign prostatic hyperplasia should use them cautiously. If you've recently had a heart attack or a stroke, suffer from hypertension, or angina, you should not take ED tablets.

The arteries may also be affected by the common but little harmful adverse effects of erectile dysfunction medication. The most frequent adverse effects comprehend surge of heat, migraine, and sinus congestion. Other side effects include backaches, indigestion, muscle soreness, and rashes.

All of these symptoms will pass, but there is a small but real risk of irreversible vision or hearing loss if it occurs suddenly.

3. Dosage and Side Effects

Viagra can produce some major negative effects. These can include a persistent erection known medically as priapism, a sudden loss of vision in one or both eyes, and a sudden decline in hearing or loss of hearing altogether. After taking Viagra, some men have reported experiencing adverse side effects such as cardiac arrest, stroke, irregular heartbeats, and even death. It was discovered that the majority of these guys, but not all of them, had heart problems before they started taking Viagra. It is not known whether Viagra was the source of these problems or whether it aggravated them.

Principal Unwanted Effects of Taking Viagra

Viagra, like any other medication, comes with its own unique set of potential adverse effects and safety concerns.

Dizziness, Headache, Flushing & Upset stomach

It is possible to experience symptoms such as nausea, flushing, headaches, and dizziness. There may also be visual alterations like increased light sensitivity, impaired vision, or difficulty distinguishing blue and green hues. Advice your physician right away if any of these negative conditions continue or get worse. As you stand up from sitting or lying down, it is essential to restrain the possibility of feeling giddiness.

Remember that the motive your physician prescribed you Viagra is that the advantages override the risks. Most people using this drug don't document any bad side effects.

Dangers to the Heart's Health

If you already have heart problems, engaging in sexual activity could potentially put your heart under further strain. If you have cardiac disease and feel any of the following dangerous adverse effects while engaging in sexual intercourse, you should immediately cease and call your doctor: extreme giddiness, light-headed, chest discomfort, or left arm dolor.

Blood pressure

Viagra and other medications like it were first developed with the intention of treating persons who suffered from pulmonary arterial hypertension, also known as high blood pressure in the arteries that supply the lungs. In point of fact, the company that makes Viagra also sells a different form of sildenafil under the brand name Revatio. This version of the medication is reserved exclusively for the therapy of PAH. Due to the fact that Viagra reduces blood pressure, it carries the chance of producing adverse effects if the blood pressure drops too low. Several of the more typical Viagra adverse effects, such as dizziness, fainting, and lightheadedness while standing, can be caused by low blood pressure, even if it is only minor. However, persons who took Viagra in conjunction with other blood pressure drugs, particularly alpha blockers, were the only ones who reported having clinically significant drops in their blood pressure as a side effect.

Sudden Vision Loss

NAION is a condition that can very rarely cause sudden vision loss in one or both eyes, including complete and permanent blindness. Ask for medical care right away and cease the consume of sildenafil if you feel this potentially fatal adverse effect. If you have heart problems, diabetes, high blood cholesterol, certain other eye disorders ("crowded disk"), increased blood pressure, are over the age of 50, or if you are a smoker, you have a slightly increased chance of having NAION. This risk is also significantly increased if you are older than 50.

Sudden Hearing Loss

In extremely rare cases, patients may have an abrupt decline in their hearing, which may be accompanied by ringing in the ears and feelings of vertigo. If you have any of these side effects, you should stop taking sildenafil and ask for medical care right away.

Priapism

This is a condition in which a man experiences an erection that continues for a number of hours, generally for more than 4 hours, despite the absence of stimulation or after the cessation of stimulation. In the event that the condition is not addressed right away, priapism might cause irreparable damage to the penis.

How long do the adverse effects typically last?

The majority of the negative effects that are frequently associated with Viagra are very transient. Due to the fact that sildenafil has a half-life of around four hours, headaches, nausea, stomach trouble, and other similar undesirable effects should disappear within approximately four to twelve hours.

Other adverse effects, like erections that are painful or last for a long time, changes in vision or hearing, severe allergic responses, stroke, or cardiovascular problems, will call for emergency medical attention. All of these factors have the potential to result in chronic problems, some of which may potentially last a lifetime. The vision impairment caused by NAION is irreversible.

In the extremely unlikely case that you experience a painful or protracted erection that lasts for more than four hours, you should immediately cease using this medication and seek medical assistance; otherwise, you run the possibility of developing irreversible difficulties.

It is quite uncommon for this drug to lead to a grave allergic reaction. Still, you must ask for instant medical care if you notice any signs of an obvious and important allergic reaction, such as skin rashes, pricking and lump (especially of the face, tongue, and throat), giddiness, and hard-ship in inspiring. These symptoms may indicate anaphy-laxis.

The appropriate amount at the appropriate time is essential

There are three different dosage levels available for Viagra: 25 milligrams mg, 50 mg, and 100 mg. In most cases, your medical provider will proceed with the dosage that is sug-gested. After that, they will make adjustments to your dos-age over time in order to find the amount that is optimal for you. In the end, your physician will prescribe the lowest possible dosage that still achieves the intended effect.

The following information provides a description of dos-ages that are typically suggested or used. However, you should make sure to assume the dose that has been sug-gested by your physician. They will provide the correct dosage for you calculated on your particular necessities.

The appropriate dose for treating erectile dysfunction

When treating erectile dysfunction (ED), the recom-mended amount of Viagra is 50 milligrams, to be taken as needed approximately one hour before sexual intercourse. You can assume it from 1.5 hour to 3.5 hours earlier than intercourse. Additionally, you must not take over one dose per day.

You should discuss the effects of the 50-mg dose with your primary care physician once you have tried it. This includes whether or not you experienced any adverse effects and whether or not your erectile function improved.

Your physician can recommend lowering your dosage of Viagra to 25 milligrams or raising it to 100 milligrams, depending on how well the drug worked for you. Alternately, they can recommend that you keep taking the same dose of 50 mg. You will carry on taking Viagra only when it is required of you. The suggested dosage is once a day at the most.

Having said that, the medication shouldn't be taken on a daily basis. Talk to your physician if you are interested in a treatment for ED that only needs to be taken once daily, such as tadalafil (Cialis).

Maximum Viagra dosage

The maximum amount of Viagra that should be used on a daily basis is 100 milligrams, and this amount should be taken just once. People that have certain medical issues or use particular medications could find that this dosage is too high for them to safely take. Therefore, it is essential that you do not take any more Viagra than what is recommended by your medical professional. Talk to your healthcare provider about the possibility of raising your dosage if the one you are now taking for your ED isn't helping very much.

Is long-term use of Viagra possible?

Yes, Viagra is often prescribed on an as-needed basis for erectile dysfunction. If you and your medical provider decide that sildenafil is a good treatment option for you, you will probably continue taking it for as long as you have ED.

Dosage adjustments

Some individuals would benefit more from a Viagra dosage that is significantly lower. This is often the result of a number of different factors, such as having a number of certain medical issues. These factors are as follows:

- Having reached the age of 65 or older

- Having kidney or liver problems

- Using a specific class of medication known as an alpha-blocker, which is prescribed for the treatment of high blood pressure or prostate illness. Examples of these drugs are Flomax, Cardura, and Minipress.

Talk to your medical provider if any of the previously mentioned events affect you. They could modify the amount of Viagra you take.

When it is not appropriate to take Viagra

If you have allergies to sildenafil citrate, you should not use this medication. If you are taking other medications to deal with PAH (pulmonary arterial hypertension), or if you are on nitrates, you should also avoid using Viagra.

Sildenafil must not be assumed by people who are simultaneously using a nitrate medication for the treatment of chest discomfort or heart diseases. Some medications, such as pentyl nitrate or nitrite, also include nitrates. Nitrates can be found in nitrite ("poppers"). Combining sildenafil with any medication that contains nitrates can result in an abrupt and potentially life-threatening hypotension.

Tell your doctor if you have or suffered from any of the following: heart problems or heart rate difficulties, coronary artery dysfunction; a cardiac arrest, collapse, or heart problems; hypotension or hypertension; hepatic or renal system disease; a bleeding problem like hemophilia; a gastric lesion; "oculus pigmentosus" (a genetic factor of the eye).

Viagra has been associated to a decrease in the bloodstream to the nervous system of the eyes, which can result in a sudden loss of vision. This has happened in a few people who have been assuming sildenafil. The majority of these individuals also suffered from cardiovascular disease, diabetes, hypertension, or excessive lipoprotein level. Additionally, people who have a tobacco addiction or are older than 45 were more likely to have experienced this side effect. There is an absence of proof to show that Viagra may be the true cause of eyesight loss.

Individuals who are also taking nitrate drugs (such as nitroglycerin) to control high blood pressure after surgery or certain cardiac diseases should avoid taking Viagra.

If you use illegal narcotics commonly referred to as "poppers," you should not use Viagra (such as amyl nitrate or amyl nitrite, and butyl nitrate). If you have ever experienced an allergic reaction to sildenafil, which is contained in Viagra and Revatio, or any of the other ingredients in Viagra, you should take any medications that are classified as guanylate cyclase stimulators.

4.   Combination with other Medications and Alcohol

Some drugs, when taken in conjunction with ED medications, have the potential to cause potentially life-threatening drops in blood pressure, which could result in a heart attack or stroke; a possibly hazardous "overdose," even when the recommended dosage is followed; and a reduction in the efficacy of the ED medications themselves.

The medications include the typical culprits, such as blood pressure medication that contains nitrates. Nitrates, when associated with Viagra, Cialis, or Levitra, have the ability to origin threatening hypotension. This fall in blood pressure could even be fatal. However, even well-known medications, such as Flomax and Provigil, as well as grapefruit juice, must not be combined with erectile dysfunction tablets. Some medications raise plasma levels of ED drugs, which can potentially lead to toxicity, whereas other medications lower plasma levels of ED medications, which renders the medications ineffective. The following are some examples:

Flomax could be a possible trigger for low blood pressure (Boehringer Ingelheim)

Grapefruit juice, Reyataz (made by Bristol-Myers Squibb), Diflucan (made by Pfizer), Gleevec (made by Novartis), Crixivan (made by Merck), Tykerb (made by GlaxoSmithKline), Mifeprex (made by Danco Labs), Viracept (made by Pfizer), and Ketek all have the potential to be hazardous (Sanofi-Aventis)

Interactions Between Viagra & Other Drugs

Drug interplay may vary the mode the medication act or increase the probability that you will experience critical side effects. This book doesn't present all of the existing drug interactions. Write about everything you utilize, such as herbaceous medicines, and provide it to your doctor. Without first talking to your doctor, you must not modify the amount of medicines, cease assuming drugs, or begin to use any unused one.

Riociguat is a product that is a potential interplay for this drug.

When used with nitrates, sildenafil can result in a dangerously low blood pressure reading for the patient. When blood pressure sinks to a threatening low degree, dizziness, fainting, and even heart attacks and strokes can occur. Sildenafil should not be taken in conjunction with any of the following: "Poppers" are a type of recreational drug that contain amyl nitrate, amyl nitrite, or butyl nitrite and are used to relieve chest pain and angina. Nitrates are utilized to deal with chest discomfort and angina pectoris.

If you are simultaneously being treated for an enlarged prostate/BPH or high blood pressure with an alpha blocker medicine (such as doxazosin or tamsulosin), your blood pressure may drop too low, which may cause you to feel dizzy or even pass out. In order to reduce the likelihood of you experiencing low blood pressure, your healthcare provider may recommend that you begin treatment with a lower dose of sildenafil.

The elimination of sildenafil might be influenced by other medications, which can have an effect on how well sildenafil works. Other examples include ketoconazole, clarithromycin, ritonavir and saquinavir, hepatitis C virus protease inhibitors (such as boceprevir and telaprevir), mifepristone and rifampin, and a number of others.

Avoid using this drug in conjunction with any other kind of medication that comprehends sildenafil citrate or any other one that treats PAH or impotence in the same way.

Interactions that are often checked

Common medications including atorvastatin, Cialis (tadalafil), gabapentin, losartan, metformin, and omeprazole had their interactions checked through studies and trials.

Other medications, such as simvastatin, tamsulosin, tramadol, and trazodone, as well as vitamins B12 (cyanocobalamin) and D3, may also be included on this list (cholecalciferol).

Alcohol's Effects on Viagra and Its Interactions

Some people drink alcohol in order to feel more relaxed before engaging in sexual activity. In addition, while having one or two drinks before engaging in sexual activity may help you get in the mood for it, drinking too much in the hours leading up to it may cause you to struggle to get an erection. People who drink a lot are at a greater risk of developing these issues, which may eventually become the norm for them.

If you already struggle with erectile dysfunction (ED), drinking alcohol probably won't make it any simpler for you to get or retain an erection. Alcohol is a sedative of the CNS and this signifies that it can decelerate the impulses that are sent between the brain cells. Since your central nervous system plays a big part in an erection, slowing down these signals could potentially cause problems with an erection.

Additionally, alcohol might have additional consequences on your health that can contribute to erectile dysfunction. This can have a number of effects, including a reduction in the amount of testosterone in your body as well as effects on your neurons, heart, and blood vessels.

Can I drink alcohol when using erectile dysfunction medication like Viagra?

As was just mentioned, drinking alcohol can potentially bring on ED or make the condition worse. Therefore, if you are using a medicine like Viagra to help you develop or keep an erection, the effectiveness of the medication could be diminished if you drink alcohol. If you are taking a medication for erectile dysfunction, it is recommended that you either cut back significantly on your alcohol usage or completely abstain from drinking alcohol.

Consuming alcohol while taking these prescriptions cannot only reduce the effectiveness of your medication, but it also has the potential to exacerbate its negative effects, such as flushing and headaches.

Is it acceptable to drink while assuming Viagra?

It's possible that some people won't have any problems if they have one or two drinks while taking drugs like Viagra. However, there are a few things about you, such as your age, other medications you're taking, and the dose that you're taking, that can make you more susceptible to either Viagra or alcohol, or even both. These things can potentially make the combination more hazardous to you. It is therefore in your best interest to consult with your healthcare professional before you even think about drinking alcohol while you are taking ED medication.

Are there any adverse effects when mixing ED medicine like Viagra with alcohol?

There is a possibility that the effects of alcohol on ED medication will be felt more strongly by certain individuals than by others who drink the same amount of alcohol. For instance, as you become older, you may become more sensitive to the effects of substances like alcohol. As was just said, drinking alcohol might increase the negative effects that Viagra causes.

It is possible that you are taking these medications during a time in your life when you are more susceptible to the negative effects of alcohol because the chance of getting erectile dysfunction increases with age. If you combine the use of alcohol and medication in this way, you run the possibility of increasing the likelihood that you will have trouble.

How does alcohol interact with medications that are utilized to deal with ED?

PDE5 inhibitors operate by preventing a protein from degrading (getting rid of) a chemical that is required for an erection. This allows for a greater quantity of the chemical to be present for a longer period of time. This causes the muscles in the penis to relax, and it also causes the blood vessels to widen (a process known as vasodilation), both of which aid enhance blood flow, which is necessary for maintaining an erection. To put it another way, having more blood in the penis improves the quality of an erection.

While drinking, your blood ducts widen, and can cause flushing of the face (redness and warmth) and migraine. This is because alcohol dilates the vessels.

Vasodilation has been associated to hypotension in some patients. Due to the potential for a reduction in blood pressure, certain drugs, such as Viagra, should not be taken in conjunction with other blood pressure medications (such alpha blockers), unless extreme caution is exercised. And because Viagra can cause potentially life-threatening decreases in blood pressure, you should avoid taking any other drugs that lower blood pressure, such as nitrates for chest discomfort. When added to the equation, alcohol has the potential to make your blood pressure readings much worse.

If you drink alcohol while taking an ED medication, you run the chance of accelerating or worsening the onset of vasodilating adverse effects.

Drinking and ED

Researchers from Loyola University examined the findings of 25 years' worth of studies on the impact of alcohol consumption on the reproductive system of men. Here are some of the findings that they obtained. These side effects are not unique to the interaction of Viagra with alcohol because they are caused by alcohol use in general. You may still want to think about how drinking affects your sexual health and performance if you have erectile dysfunction.

Implications for both testosterone and estrogen levels

The levels of testosterone and estrogen can be impacted by both one-time heavy drinking episodes and persistent alcohol use. The testes of a man are the organs responsible for producing testosterone. It is implicated in many of the body's processes and operations. Additionally, it is the hormone that is most closely associated with male sexuality, and it is the hormone that is accountable for the development of sexual organs as well as sperm.

Estrogen is a hormone that is primarily found in females, but it can also be found in males. It is connected to the maturation of female sexual traits as well as the process of reproduction.

If you are a man and consume more than a moderate amount of alcohol, it may cause your testosterone levels to drop while simultaneously increasing your estrogen levels. It's possible that your body will become more feminine if you have low testosterone levels and high estrogen levels. Either your breasts or your body hair could start to grow out.

The consequences for the testicles

Consuming alcohol can be harmful to the testicles. According to some sources, drinking a lot of alcohol over time can lead your testicles to get smaller. Both the amount and the grade of your sperm will suffer as a result of this.

Influences on the male reproductive organ

Abuse of alcohol may be connected with prostatitis, according to the findings of several sources (inflammation of the prostate gland). The patient may experience pain, edema, and difficulty urinating as symptoms of this condition. There is a potential relationship between soreness of the prostate gland and ED.

After taking my prescription for ED, how soon until I may start drinking again?

It is in your best interest to refrain from consuming alcohol until all of the medication has been eliminated from your system. Cialis has been shown to have a half-life of up to five days, whereas Viagra and Levitra have a half-life of approximately one day. However, because each person's physical make-up is unique, it is in your best interest to consult with your doctor regarding the appropriate timing for you to start drinking again.

It is important to keep in mind that pharmaceuticals for sex, such as Viagra, should only be used when necessary and not on a regular basis. For this reason, it is not always predictable to anticipate when you will take the medication. Because of this, if you have already had a few drinks, you should probably give taking medicine for erectile dysfunction a second thought before doing so.

It is highly recommended that you abstain from drinking alcohol while you are on ED drugs such as Viagra: not only can alcohol nullify the advantages of the drug, but it also has the potential to exacerbate its negative side effects, such as flushing and headaches.

If you are assuming drugs such as Viagra at the moment, you need to talk to your doctor before consuming any alcohol. Alterations to your way of life, as well as potential underlying causes and other ED treatment choices, may be brought up at your appointment with your healthcare physician.

5.   Different Ways of Treating Erectile Dysfunction

What transpires in the bedroom is typically kept in the bedroom, except for when things are going awry in the bedroom. Male erectile dysfunction has become the most prevalent medical issue that men seek treatment for. Oral medications like "the blue pill" or one of its near cousins are recommended to men the most frequently.

Oral drugs aren't the only option for treating erectile dysfunction, and they can have unpleasant side effects. Finally, some guys are unable to benefit from these drugs at all. The positive aspect is that there are different treatment options for ED.

Surgical Treatments

When a severe pelvic injury damages the penile blood vessels, it is common for males under the age of 40 to undergo Microsurgical Penile Revascularization (a surgical treatment intended to cure erectile dysfunction). Restoring blood supply to the penis with microsurgical revascularization may help these men's erections in the long run.

Surgeons can surgically bypass clogged arteries in the penis by joining one artery in the lower abdomen to one on top of the penis during this treatment, which is carried out under general anesthesia in the hospital. An erection can only be sustained if there is enough bloodstream to the penis.

If a guy has atherosclerosis, the arteries in his penis may be permanently damaged, and as a result, this surgery is not recommended for him.

Vacuum Erection Device (VED)

A vacuum erection device is a cylindrical Tube that is wrapped around the penis to help pump more blood until an erection is achieved. This is one of the first and most effective therapies for erectile dysfunction. Erectile dysfunction drugs are often used as a last resort when they fail.

After dousing your penis with oil, you put the tubing that connects your vacuum to it, and you're ready for action! For an erection to occur, you have to manually pump on a vacuum device until the air has been expelled from the tube. A constrictive band is then set round the lowest part of the penis to maintain the erection in place for up to 25/30 minutes during intercourse. The erection is gone after the band is removed following sexual contact.

Light bruising on the penis may occur as a side effect, however, this normally does not cause any discomfort and usually disappears within a few days.

Penile Prostheses

Vacuums and other medical devices can have a negative impact on a man's ability to express himself spontaneously. A penile prothesis—a mechanized tool put in the penis—may be recommended by doctors in this situation.

This can be done for men who suffer from erectile dysfunction due to the signs and symptoms of type 2 diabetes, heart illness, or a spinal cord injury. A man's capacity to orgasm or ejaculate will not be negatively affected by any of the two types of implants.

Malleable Implants

Surgically implanted mechanical devices give long-term hardness to the penis with malleable penile implants. An incision is performed near the underside of the penis, and an aperture is made in the two lengthy ducts of springy tissue that compose the rod of the spermatic cord. Each opening is replenished with a semi-inflexible bar. There is an anesthetic used throughout the surgery, which lasts between 30 and 60 minutes. You may be able to get out of the clinic the very same day as your procedure.

Your doctor may recommend that you refrain from sexual activities for at least 6 weeks following surgery, and could also prescribe pain meds if necessary. In comparison to inflatable implants, these ones are easier to spot because of their constant firmness. In order to hide this, the implanted rods can be bent downwards by hand.

Implants That Inflate

Erections that are reliable, hard, and spontaneous can be achieved with inflatable penile implants that can be inflated to mimic the sensation of having an erection and then deflated after the sexual act. It takes one to two hours for the implant to be installed in the penis and scrotum, which contains two inflatable cylinders, the reservoir, and the pump unit. It is possible to inflate the prosthesis and achieve a "erection-like" state by pressing the pump part of the device into the scrotum, which is located near the bladder.

Having the penile prosthesis surgically implanted will require anesthesia and a recovery period of four to six weeks, during which time your doctor may suggest you to refrain from having sexual relations. Depending on the extent of their recovery, some men can go home the same day as their operation, while others will need to stay in the hospital overnight. Following surgery, patients may be provided pain medication as needed.

Because inflatable implants are mechanical, they will eventually wear out. For example, surgery may be necessary if this happens.

Injections into the Vernacular Veins (ICI)

However, unsettling the thought may be, a drug injected into the penis is significantly more effective at increasing blood flow than any medicine taken orally could be. A thin needle is utilized to provide the medication to the man's penis. This is an injection that you give yourself, but doctors usually show patients how to do it right and give the first shot in the clinic.

Side effects of this therapy include mild pain or bleeding at the site of injection, an erection that lasts longer than desired, and the formation of scar tissue in the underlying tissue of the penis, which happens mostly in people who use this therapy for a long time.

Natural remedies

Natural ED therapies are widely accessible; however, none has been approved by the FDA. Due to the lack of regulatory oversight, the FDA does not endorse over-the-counter (OTC) medicines for erectile dysfunction. Unknown substances, improper quantities of prescription medications, or different doses of components than the label implies are common in these items.

According to the Urology Care Foundation, which is in agreement with this point of view, the use of supplements, despite their widespread popularity and the fact that they are frequently less expensive than prescription medications, does not ensure that they are safe or effective. Erectile dysfunction natural therapies have received relatively little research. From moderate to severe, many medicines have side effects.

It was also determined that four popular herbal medications used to treat ED were not properly monitored and could pose a public health risk. There is a necessity for exhaustive investigation and surveillance, according to the scientists.

L-arginine

One of the essential amino acids is L-arginine. It is a vasodilator, which signifies that it can assist in widening the arteries. A theoretical raise in bloodstream to the penis could lead to erections, at least theoretically. ED and low L-arginine levels were found to be associated in a study published in 2017.

It hasn't been established, however, that L-arginine pills can help with ED. This remedy's safety and efficacy will have to wait for further investigation.

Prescription ED medicines, such as Viagra, and L-arginine should not be taken together since they can produce dangerously low blood pressure. Headaches and flushes are also possible side effects.

L-arginine may cause nausea, abdominal cramps, hypotension, and a raise in lipid levels, among other side effects.

Propionyl-L-carnitine

Men with ED and diabetes who took propionyl-L-carnitine in addition to sildenafil saw greater results than those who took sildenafil just. Still, additional investigation is required to determine the therapy's security and usefulness.

There are normally just moderate side effects like itching, rashes, nausea, and heartburn. People with vascular illness, increased blood pressure, diabetes, or liver cirrhosis should avoid using this substance altogether.

Dehydroepiandrosterone

DHEA, a precursor of sex hormones such as testosterone and estrogen, aids in the production of these hormones. Natural DHEA levels fall with age, which could lead to diminished sexual performance. Supplementing with DHEA may help some men with erectile dysfunction, although others have found zero evidence to support this.

When DHEA is used orally in the authorized doses, there are little side effects. There is the chance of experiencing negative effects, such as lethargy, headaches, and acne.

Ginkgo

It's possible that ginkgo biloba could promote sexual desire and combat ED by enhancing blood flow to the penis. NCCIH, on the other hand, argues that there is no evidence that ginkgo can help with any health condition, including Alzheimer's and Parkinson's disease.

Constipation and diarrhea are some of the negative effects of utilizing it. It is also possible for it to raise the chance of bleeding, which can make it potentially hazardous for individuals who are using blood thinners like warfarin (Coumadin) or who suffer from other bleeding problems.

Ginseng

Popular home cure Panax ginseng, or Ginseng: this plant's compounds may assist relax the body's smooth muscles, which could aid in obtaining an erection. Although a study published in 2012 revealed that extract from ginseng berries could help cure mild to moderate erectile dysfunction (ED), additional high-quality research is required to confirm this.

Insomnia is the most prevalent complication of ginseng use. Low or high blood pressure and headaches are also potential adverse reactions.

Yohimbine

The traditional aphrodisiac yohimbine is derived from the cortex of an African tree. Yohimbine from tree cortex has not been proven to treat ED, according to the NCCIH. One kind of yohimbine, known as yohimbine hydrochloride, is available by prescription only for the treatment of erectile dysfunction (ED). This is a distinct product from tree bark-based dietary supplements.

Research shows that yohimbine can cause major adverse effects like heart attacks and convulsions. Some of the other adverse effects include stomach pains, nervousness, and high blood pressure.

Horny goat weed

Horny goat weed, or Epimedium grandiflorum, is a traditional treatment for boosting fertility. In treating erectile dysfunction brought on by nerve injury, a component of horny goat weed, icariin, showed promise in a 2010 research. Researchers, on the other hand, did this investigation on rats whose nerves had been damaged and on lab-grown nerve cells.

Although this supplement is generally well-tolerated, there isn't enough data to recommend it for regular consumption. Vomiting, heart palpitations, and dry mouth are all possible side effects.

Participating in regular physical activity

Emotional and physical well-being can be improved via regular exercise. It's an amazing way to better your general health.

A balanced diet

Eating well helps to maintain the health of the circulatory system as well as the rest of the body. Consume a diet rich in fruits, greens, grains and cereals, and protein to lower your risk of heart disease, artery clogs, obesity, and diabetes.

Smoking and drinking should be reduced

Due to its effect on blood flow, smoking is an important risk factor for ED. The excessive consumption of alcoholic beverages might also have a detrimental effect. As stated by the CDC, men ought to restrict alcohol use up to 2 drinks daily and women to 1 drink daily.

Decrease tension

Both the desire to have sexual encounters and the ability to maintain an erection can be significantly impacted by stress and worry. Many factors can be a fount of tension.

Medicines Taken Orally

There are several different types of ED drugs that work by increasing the quantity of nitric oxide in the organism, which helps to relax the muscles of the penis. You can have an erection in reaction to sexual excitation as a result of this.

6. Bonus Chapter: Frequently Asked Questions

Is it hard to get Viagra Prescription?

When talking about getting a Rx for Viagra, it's usually not that tough. If you suffer from erectile dysfunction, your doctor may prescribe Viagra if they believe it is a safe and effective treatment for your condition, given your symptoms, medical history, and current state of health.

Why was Viagra invented?

Viagra was first made by Pfizer to treat high blood pressure (hypertension) and chest pain (angina pectoris). Researchers found that the medicine was more effective at causing erections than curing angina during heart clinical studies.

Is taking Viagra safe?

In a nutshell, Viagra is completely risk-free. To ensure its safety, the medicine is manufactured by Pfizer, a well-known pharmaceutical corporation. The medicine will not damage you if you use it as suggested and attend the instructions.

What is the indicated age for taking Viagra?

18+ years.

What are the risks of assuming Viagra and generic Viagra?

Some individuals may suffer from giddiness, migraine, flushing, or stomach aches. Vision alterations, such as impaired vision, increased light sensitivity, or difficulty distinguishing between blue and green, may also develop. Talk to your doctor or chemist right away if any of these symptoms continue or get worse.

Does Viagra work without a prostate?

Impotence in men who have had their prostate removed can be treated with Viagra. The medicine boosts erection performance by about 60% in men with intact nerves, whereas this rises to only 20% in men without nerves.

Does Viagra create an addiction?

Sildenafil's efficacy and safety have been deemed satisfactory. Sildenafil is not addictive or habit-forming when taken for short or long periods of time.

Is it possible to overdose on Viagra?

Overdosing on the medication might result in dangerously high amounts of the substance in the body. Low blood pressure is one of the potential negative reactions of using an immoderate quantity of this drug.

What is recommended Viagra dosage?

For people between the ages of 18 and 64, 50 mg is the suggested dosage. People over the age of 65 are more likely to begin taking 25 mg than those under the age of 65. Based on how effective and well tolerated the drug is, the dosage could be increased to 100 mg.

Can it be harmful if a man takes Viagra when it is not really needed?

Viagra and similar drugs should not be taken without a doctor's supervision. Illegal drugs may be contaminated or have negative effects that could lead to an increased chance of acquiring ED. If antidepressants are the source of their sexual dysfunction, some men may find that taking Viagra increases their sexual desire.

Does Viagra affect the kidney?

Sudden hearing loss & prolonged erections that damage the penis are two rare but dangerous side effects. On one occasion, a patient suffered an acute kidney injury as a result of using Viagra.

Can heart patients take Viagra?

Preliminary studies have demonstrated that this medication is safe for patients with a steady cardiac situation.

Is it fine to assume Viagra every day?

Yes, sildenafil, the generic variant of Viagra, can be taken every day.

How many times a day may I assume Viagra?

Just once. Never use it more than once daily without talking with your doctor.

Is it risky to assume Viagra in your youth?

In the case of young men who are really anxious or distressed about having sex, it is acceptable.

What's the strongest dosage of Viagra taken at one time?

100 mg but not everyone has the capacity to tolerate such a dosage. Always consult your doctor for the recommended dosage.

Is natural Viagra effective for men?

Some herbal or natural Viagra products may help with ED by loosening the walls of the blood vessels, which enhances the flow of blood. This supplement, however, can induce very low blood pressure because the dosage of the plants it contains is not prescribed.

Can Viagra help people who had prostate surgery?

Yes. Men who have had their prostate removed can benefit from the use of Viagra as a treatment for impotence.

Is Viagra safe for Hypertensive Patients?

Viagra and other ED medications, such as Stendra, Cialis, and Levitra, are safe, effective, and acceptable for many people with hypertension.

What other symptoms do people use Viagra for?

In addition to treating erectile dysfunction (ED), pulmonary hypertension is now another condition for which Viagra is prescribed. According to a recent report, the medicine may also be helpful in dealing with many other sicknesses.

Is there a herbal supplement that works like Viagra?

According to some experts, an amino acid called L-citrulline may have similar effects as Viagra. Another amino acid which has been demonstrated to enhance blood flow is L-arginine, which this amino acid serves as a precursor to.

Should I use Sildenafil before or after eating?

Viagra works best if you haven't eaten before assuming it.

Can a healthy person use Viagra for more pleasure?

It is not advisable. Viagra, just like any other drug should not be taken for recreation.

How long does it take to work?

You must use sildenafil at least 1 hour before planning sexual intercourse in order to get the most out of the drug's effects.

What are the good alternatives for men suffering from ED?

Natural remedies, surgical treatments, implants, a balanced diet, and physical fitness are some of the better alternatives to ED prescription drugs.

Made in United States
North Haven, CT
13 October 2022

25343710R00046